Petals of Healing

A Guided Grief Journal

This journal belongs to:

____

____

____

Table of Contents

Introduction

I loved my dad's hands. They were so soft and always warm, no matter how cold it was outside. As a child, I would hold his hand every chance I got. On a rainy Wednesday just a few days before my best friend's wedding four years ago, surrounded by several life-saving machines, I held my dad's hand as it went cold for the first and last time.

The grief hit immediately with the force of a truck. It was powerful, all-consuming, and both physically and emotionally excruciating. In that moment, I wondered the same thing so many other people do after a loved one dies: How am I going to live without them?

Grief is a fickle beast. Even if you see it coming in the distance, it is a giant wave that crashes with unexpected strength. It tosses you around until you accept the loss of control, letting each wave wash over you until it eventually passes. But, despite feeling unbearable, I've learned that grief is survivable.

Writing has become a time when I can feel my dad's presence instead of isolating myself in his absence. It's the act of creating which I can release emotions that have nowhere else to go. Expressing myself verbally has never come easy to me, but through the hundreds of poems I've written since losing my dad, I've gained a sense of empowerment at a time that has otherwise made me feel so powerless. Writing gives me a sense of control, especially during times where I've felt like I didn't have any.

Step by step, I'm charting a new path for myself after losing my dad, one that is so painful but propelling me forward. By facing my sorrow head on, I created an opportunity to remember and reconnect with him. Maybe I can't hide from the grief. But, thankfully, I can write through it and so can you.

Welcome to Petals of Healing.

This guided grief journal was designed with love, to help you heal after the loss of a loved one. In these pages are poems, exercises, techniques, affirmations, writing prompts and space to journal through your grief journey.

What I learned about grief is there is no destination. Grief is multilayered and one of those layers is allowing yourself to heal. I hope this book offers you comfort and a place to remember the person who died, a place to tell your story and explore your grief.

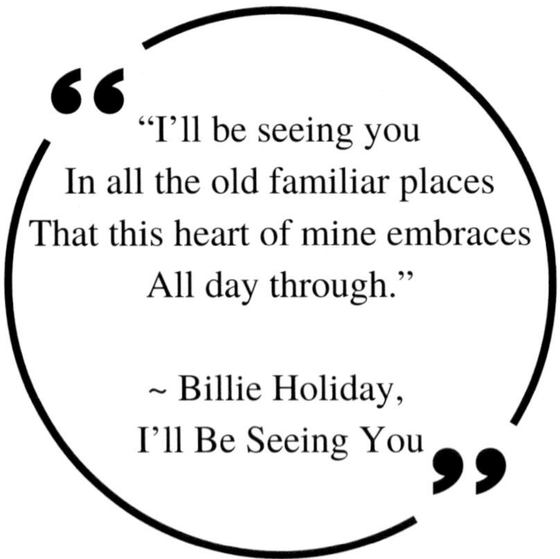

Grief is our response to the love we have for our loved ones. It helps connect us to our past; it bonds us with others through our compassion, and it helps provide perspective for finding strength in the darkest of times.

There is no rule book on grief, no checklist. Grief is something that we just have to allow into our lives and work through on our terms. All grief journeys are valid and true - because they are YOUR truth. There is no right and wrong way to grieve, there's only your way. Your journey will have stops and starts. Sometimes you'll find you spend months stuck in one place and that's normal. After all, you are not just grieving the death of a person, which is agonizing, but you are also grieving the loss of who and how you were in your relationships and in the world.

We need to own the right to feel grief and for everyone to acknowledge, it's quite normal. Yes, it's scary and messy and yes, it can't be easily controlled, but we need to acknowledge that grief is the price we pay for love. Grief is part of existing in the world and is as real as any other part of life, as real as love, hope, and joy. Remember that no one emotion is more right or valid than another, but understanding what you are feeling can be important in helping identify what you may need at a particular time.

Grief is never experienced the same way for any two people. But it helps to know that grief impacts most of us in a way where the pain is intense at the beginning, but the frequency (if not the intensity) of the pain lessens over time.

Grief is personal. Loss can leave us feeling isolated and vulnerable. For some, mourning is a new experience, whereas, for others, it is a familiarity they have known before. Everyone has had their own experiences with grief and with the loss it has caused them.

Grief is one of the most powerful emotions we experience as humans and it can be very difficult to discuss a loss with others. Writing is a tried and trusted method for helping us come to terms with the intense and often overwhelming sorrow we feel at the death of a loved one.
This journal offers you some guidance, while giving you plenty of space to grieve in your own way and explore what you are feeling.

 The tools inside of this book can help you process your loss and move forward in your grief. This is not to imply that you "let go" or "move on." You will always love the one you lost! But we do need to both mourn our loss and continue to live.

Grief journaling is not about writing perfectly. It's important to remember:

- This is your book and there is no right or wrong way to use it.
- Mindfully engage with your whole being.
- Approach familiar subjects as if it were the first time.
- Walk up to the edge, but don't fall over.
- Seek out physical and emotional support as needed.

Understanding grief and finding you are not alone in your feelings as you use each exercise will help you train and thereby gentle-down your grief. The eventual goal, in your own time and in your own way, is to develop a relational home for your grief. I cannot promise that your grief will go away or even that you will want it to, but with time and practice, you will learn to let grief inspire you rather than deaden you.

I will reach out for support when I need it.

Stages of Grief

We've all heard about the "stages" of grief. In fact, if you're like me, you've probably had those stages used against you along your grief journey because you're not "trying to move ahead," or "you're taking too long."

The five stages of the grief model were developed by Elisabeth Kübler-Ross, and became famous after she published her book *On Death and Dying* in 1969. Kübler-Ross developed this model to describe people with terminal illness facing their own death. But we soon adapted it as a way of thinking about our grief in general.

The five stages — denial, anger, bargaining, depression and acceptance — are often talked about as if they happen in order, moving from one stage to the next. You might hear people say things like 'Oh, I've moved on from denial and now I think I'm entering the anger stage.' But this isn't often the case.

Kübler-Ross, in her writing, clarifies that the stages are non-linear–people can experience these aspects of grief at different times and they do not happen in any order. You might not experience all the stages, and you might find feelings are quite different from the ones in her model.

"The reality is that you will grieve forever. You will not 'get over' the loss of a loved one; you will learn to live with it. You will heal and you will rebuild yourself around the loss you have suffered. You will be whole again but you will never be the same again.
Nor should you be the same nor would you want to."

— Elisabeth Kübler-Ross

Though the five stages of grief may be the most widely known, there's now enough evidence to create other versions, such as the seven stages of grief and loss. These seven stages of grief reflect the process of all types of loss.

Shock & Denial - The self-defense stage of the mind. A massive blow, sending us into a state of shock, paralysis, and numbness. The fact that you have experienced a loss is evident now, but you still have underlying feelings of shock. A detachment from your current reality.

Pain & Guilt - As the shock wears off, it is replaced with the suffering of unbelievable pain. Grief makes you feel out of control. You may have guilty feelings or remorse over things you did or didn't say or do with your loved one.

Anger & Bargaining - The what if and if only stage? The trying to explain the things that could have gone differently. "What if we had that second opinion?" "If only we could have taken him/her to the hospital sooner." Frustration gives way to anger, and you may lash out and lay unwarranted blame for the death on someone else. You may rail against fate, questioning, "Why me?" You may also try to bargain in vain with the powers that be for a way out of your despair.

Depression, Reflection & Loneliness - This is often around the time your friends and family may think you should be getting on with your life. A long period of sad reflection will likely take over. As your panic begins to subside, the emotional fog begins to lift, the loss feels more present. In those moments, you tend to pull inward as the sadness grows. You might find yourself avoiding people, reaching out less to others about what you are going through.

The Upward Turn - As you start to adjust to life without your loved one, your life becomes a little calmer. Your physical symptoms lessen, and your "depression" begins to lift slightly. This is the part of the grieving process that you'll start to see the light a bit at the end of the tunnel. It's a middle ground of all the grief symptoms that you'll go through but it's one that you can build upon.

Reconstruction & Working Through - As you become more functional, your mind starts working again, and you find yourself seeking realistic solutions to problems posed by life without your loved one. You start to work on reconstructing yourself and your life without them.

Acceptance & Hope - Acceptance does not mean that you no longer think about your loved ones. During this, the last of the seven stages in this grief model, you learn to accept and deal with the reality of your situation. Acceptance does not necessarily mean instant happiness. Given the pain and turmoil you have experienced, you can never return to the carefree, untroubled YOU that existed before this loss. But you will find a way forward. You will start to look forward and plan things for the future.

"You will lose someone you can't live without, and your heart will be badly broken, and the bad news is that you never completely get over the loss of your beloved. But this is also the good news. They live forever in your broken heart that doesn't seal back up. And you come through. It's like having a broken leg that never heals perfectly – that still hurts when the weather gets cold, but you learn to dance with the limp."

— Anne Lamott

Grief Assessment

Check all that apply:

- ◯ I have someone that I can talk with about my feelings.

- ◯ I can express my feelings openly.

- ◯ The loss has become a reality now.

- ◯ I am sleeping enough at this time.

- ◯ I am not self-medicating with alcohol.

- ◯ My appetite is back to normal.

- ◯ I do not avoid people or isolate myself for extended periods of time.

- ◯ As time passes, I am coping better.

- ◯ I am not concerned about where I am in the grieving process.

- ◯ I have made peace with my loss.

- ◯ I am no longer angry about my loss.

- ◯ My sadness lifts at times.

- ◯ I can remember the good times with my lost loved one.

- ◯ I want to move forward but never forget.

- ◯ I feel hopeful about the future.

The Ball in the Box

I came across 'The Ball and the Box' analogy on Twitter last year and wanted to share it with you. In her tweet, Lauren Herschel said, "So grief is like this. There's a box with a ball in it. And a pain button."

"In the beginning, the ball is huge. You can't move the box without the ball hitting the pain button. It rattles around on its own in there and hits the button over and over. You can't control it - it just keeps hurting. Sometimes it seems unrelenting."

"Over time, the ball gets smaller. It hits the button less and less, but when it does, it hurts just as much. It's better because you can function day to day more easily. But the downside is that the ball randomly hits the button when you least expect it."

"For most people, the ball never really goes away. It might hit less and less and you have more time to recover between hits, unlike when the ball was still giant."

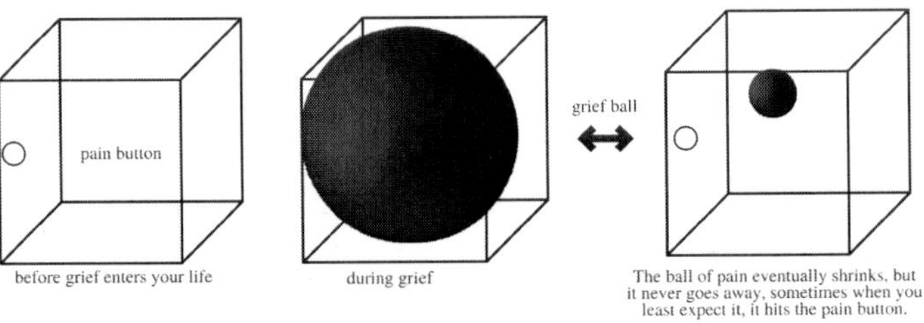

The "Ball and the Box' explains why faced with a new loss, we still experience pain for a past loss. Besides the new giant ball, the older grief ball is still bouncing around, hitting the pain button occasionally, especially when it's bouncing against the giant ball that's occupying so much of the box. This section is as much for you as it is for your friends, family, and co-workers. Most of us walk through life, carrying our own box with a ball of grief inside of it. I encourage you to share this analogy with your loved ones.

Grief Rituals

Change can be difficult and there's nothing more life-changing than losing a loved one—and the closer you were to them, the more affected you'll feel.

Over time, rituals can also help us complete one of the most important tasks of mourning — moving on with our lives and coming to terms with a loss. They can be done just once, every year on the anniversary of the loss, or simply when the emotions of grief come up. Some people do rituals on the deceased person's birthday or an anniversary. Others choose daily or weekly rituals. The frequency is a personal choice, and the style can be as elaborate or simple as you decide.

A ritual is any action done with a purpose to connect us to something or someone else. This can encompass something that is bigger than ourselves — such as religious rituals or actions that connect us to a particular person or tradition. We may not realize it, but we do mini-rituals every day already — from our morning routines of making coffee and making the bed, to brushing our teeth at night.

Rituals provide us with meaning, structure, and connectedness, which provides a healthy way to process grief, honor someone you've lost, and reconnect with them and the memories you have. Memorial services and funerals are common grief rituals that people plan and use for the loss of a loved one, but there are several other things that can be done in addition to these services to help with grief.

"If someone describes a griever to me by saying, 'Oh, she's so strong and together; she's handling her grief really well,' that's when I worry. I think someone is handling her grief well if I hear that 'she's terribly upset, she's crying constantly, she's falling apart.' Emotion isn't the problem . . . it's the natural response and the ultimate solution."
—Ashley Davis Bush

Grief Healthy Rituals

Whatever ritual you choose, do what feels comfortable for you and remain open to whatever feelings and emotions come up. Complete the following to identify some healthy rituals.

IDEA: Develop a photo album or scrapbook of pleasant memories to view when you want to remember your loved one.

List some memories here that you would include:

1

2

3

4

5

6

Establish a ritual for anniversaries, birthdays, holidays and other times. This might include a visit to the cemetery, flowers by the urn, planting a tree, placing a special rock or other symbolic token on the headstone, a special toast at holiday dinners, etc.

List some ideas below:

Some people establish a trust or memorial to fund scholarships or contribute to their favorite charity in the name of their lost loved one. Alternatively, you might recommend that people donate money to a specific fund or charity. List some ideas below:

Grief Roadblocks

When someone you love dies, everything changes.

Anger, guilt and regret are common roadblocks, and manifest differently for different people. Anger can be at — our loved one for leaving us; the medical profession for not doing more; at friends and family for not being more supportive; God for letting it happen. Guilt is often at not having done more — encouraging our loved one to take better care; guilt at not preventing a drug overdose. "If only we had done more, they'd still be here". Regret for not saying "I love you" more often; not spending more time; not apologizing.

The list goes on, but the important thing is to consider why we hold on to these emotions.

Once we understand the "why", the next step is to redirect our thinking and our energy to how we can let go of these emotions and move past the roadblock.

"One of the most important things I've learned is how deeply you can keep loving someone after they die. You may not be able to hold them or talk to them, and you may even date or love someone else, but you can still love them every bit as much."
- Sheryl Sandberg

Sometimes things are left unsaid, or issues are not resolved before the loss of a loved one. This can make it more difficult to move through grief.

- If you could speak with your loved one again, what would you like to say?

- What unresolved issues do you have that need to be addressed.

- What can you do to address any unresolved issues? (Express your gratitude to a family member, etc.)

- Often writing a letter expressing your feelings and/or thoughts can be theraputic. Read it aloud to yourself, another person, or an empty chair. (go to page 95 when you're ready to write them a letter.)

I can hold onto love and let go of grief.

Letting Go

Letting go is probably one of the hardest things to do, but with patience and practice, we can continue to find some acceptance of the idea that we had no control over what happened. Stop here, and take a moment with that. You had no control over what happened. **Repeat that to yourself**, "I had no control of what happened." Do this until the weight and burden you have been carrying has been lifted from you. By letting go, we can realize that no amount of sleepless nights or overthinking or second guessing will ever, ever, ever change what has happened. *The only thing we truly have power over is this moment - and this moment only.*

Complete the following:

- In order to fully mourn my loss, I'm letting go of these thoughts: For example: I don't want to live without him/her.

- In order to fully mourn my loss, I will let go of this guilt:

- In order to fully mourn my loss, I let go of these plans for the future:

- In order to fully mourn my loss, I will let go of these painful memories:

- In order to fully mourn my loss, I will let go of these lost opportunities:

Self-Care While Grieving

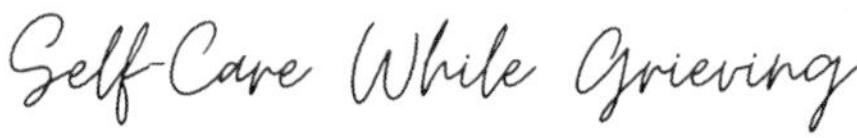

Self-care is a crucial part of the healing process and can help ease the suffering of the mind, body, and spirit. As every individual's grief is unique, so is their path to healing from a loss. What works for someone else may not work for you and that's okay. Find what self-care tips work for you. The following self-care tips are meant to assist you and give you useful tools for navigating through the ups and downs of grief.

Find ways to express your grief.
What you do is going to depend on your personality. For some, it's helpful to go into the backyard and garden or spend time at the batting cages hitting the balls over and over again. For others, creative expression is helpful. Many times, creative writing, journaling, painting, drawing, arts & crafts, or other types of self-expression help you make sense of the seemingly senseless feelings that are going on inside of you. And if you are a person of faith, prayer, meditation, or worship, these activities can help you express your grief too.

Take time to talk about your grief.
Sometimes it's helpful to talk with a safe person about the emotions swirling around inside you. If you aren't much of a talker or aren't ready to be vulnerable with someone, write your thoughts down. However, if talking to friends and family simply isn't working, then consider the benefits of a grief counselor. Sometimes the grief we feel is so incredibly deep that we need help getting back onto solid ground. If that's you, it's okay. *You are not alone.*

Take care of yourself.
Most people feel more tired and less energetic when they are grieving. For this reason, it's important to practice self-care and get plenty of sleep. If you are having trouble sleeping, stay hydrated, limit your caffeine intake, and try to make your bedroom as relaxing as possible. Additionally, eat healthy foods and participate in some kind of physical activity on a regular basis.

Cultivate an attitude of gratitude.

During times of grief, we often turn our focus inward. While this tendency is natural, it may also lead to feelings of isolation and intense focus on the loss we have suffered. Cultivating a lifestyle of self-care and gratitude can help you better process a loss by moving your eyes beyond your pain, allowing you to see the good things in life that still remain. Gratitude increases positive emotions and overall well-being, improves sleep, and fosters resilience.

Be kind to yourself.

Grief can be cruel. Give yourself the love and respect you deserve. Talk kindly to yourself and allow yourself to grieve in the time and ways that you need. Give yourself words of encouragement. Don't let your own mind hurt you further. Reflect on meaningful ways to show yourself kindness.

Allow yourself to really feel.

Feel what you need to feel. There is no right or wrong feeling during grief. You may feel numb, angry, empty, depressed, confused, etc. You may also feel relief, comfort, joy, etc. Whatever you're feeling is okay.

Permission Slip	Check off all that apply
☐	Sit with your sadness
☐	Cry
☐	Scream
☐	Have a pity part
☐	Be angry
☐	Stay in bed all day
☐	Throw things

I will
be
gentle
with
myself.

It is important to take care yourself when mourning the loss of a loved one. Use the space below to identify some ways you can do this.

To care for my physical well being, I can:

1

2

3

4

5

To care for my spiritual well being, I can:

1

2

3

4

5

To care for my emotional well being, I can:

1

2

3

4

5

To care for my mental well being, I can:

1

2

3

4

5

Positive Memories

It can be helpful in the grieving process to recall fond memories of your loved one. Use the following prompts to list the details of as many positive memories as possible.

- I remember the first time we. . .

- Our first. . .

- Our favorite place was. . .

- Our favorite meal was. . .

- The most exciting thing we did together was. . .

- The most sacred thing we did together was. . .

- Our favorite vacation spot was. . .

- Favorite pastime . . .

- We found the best place to. . .

- Our home was. . .

- His/Her hobby was. . .

- She/he always wanted to. . .

- We talked about. . .

- We loved. . .

- His/Her dream was. . .

- My favorite gift was. . .

- His/Her favorite authors were. . .

- His/Her favorite movies/shows were. . .

- We always tried to. . .

About My Grief

"Some things cannot be fixed; they can only be carried. Grief like yours, love like yours, can only be carried."
– Megan Devine

WHAT HAS BEEN CONFUSING....	WHAT HAS BEEN SURPRISING...

WHAT I HAVE BEEN THANKFUL FOR DURING MY GRIEF

MEANINGFUL OR COMFORTING QUOTE DURING MY GRIEF

My
grief
matters.

Poetry Prompts

Sadness often gives birth to the most poetical literary pieces because many people have experienced grief, or unhappiness at a certain point in their life. Write about the cause for your sadness.

Write a poem about the fondest memory you have of the person who has passed away. Why is this memory so special? How did you feel when this person died?

Death is often personified. Write a poem addressing death as a person. What is it that you would like to tell him/her? What would you want to ask them?

Write a poem about the death of a pet. What did you do to help you deal with the loss?

Write a poem about the first time you understood the concept of death.

In this section you will find a word bank and poems from two of my poetry books *Metamorphosis - A Collection of Haiku Poetry on Love, Grief and Healing* and *Life Interrupted.*

Use them along with the above prompts to help you write your own poems.

Emotions & Feelings Word Bank

abandoned, ache, adjustments, affect, aftermath, aggrieved, agony, anger, anguish, annoyed, anxious, apathetic, ashamed, awkward, avoidance, awareness, awful, baffled, bereaved, black, blame, bleak, breakdown, burden, bitter, bothered, calm, caring, churn, clasp, closure, collapse, comfort, compassion, comprehension, concerned, consequence, confident, confused, console, contempt, coping, counsel, crisis, cross, culpability, dealing with, denial, deplore, depression, deprivation, despair, despondent, devastated, devotion, dignity, dire, disbelief, discouraged, distraction, distress, discontented, disdain, disgruntled, down, downhearted, eerie, effect, embarrassed, embrace, emotional, empty, empathize, enduring, engulf, eternal, enraged, exhaustion, envious, fatal, fearful, feelings, forsaken, foolish, forgiving, frustrated, furious, gnawing, grasping, gratitude, gloomy, grateful, grief, guilt, hallowed, hardships, haunted, healing, heartbroken, heartfelt, heaven, helpless, humanity, horrified, hurt, illness, impact, impulsive, incapacitated, incoherent, in awe, inadequate, insecure, inspired, insulted, irritated, jaded, jealous, keepsake, lament, linger, livid, lonely, lost, love, loved, low, melancholy, memories, mercy, miffed, miserable, messed-up, motivated, mourn, nauseous, nervous, nightmare, numb, obligation, observe, offended, outbursts, overburdened, outcome, overcome, overjoyed, overwhelmed, paranoid, peace, petrified, perseverance, personal, perspective, petrified, pissed off, pressured, proud, poignant, preoccupied, privacy, problems, quake, quiet, quiver, ramifications, reaction, reality, receptive, recollection, recovery, reflective, regret, rejected, regroup, relationships, relentless, remember, remorse, repercussions, resilience, resent, resolve, respect, response, results, ritual, sad, salvage, satisfied, scared, scornful, self-assured, self-conscious, sensitive, serene, shame, shattered, shock, solace, somber, sorrow, strain, stressed, strong, strung-out, stupid, suicidal, support, support group, survival, survivor, surprised, suspicious, sympathy, tears, tearful, temper, terrified, terror, thankful, therapeutic, therapy, threatened, tired, trapped, trauma, traumatized, troubled, trusting, turmoil, uncomfortable, unexpected, uneasy, unspeakable, unstable, upset , urgent, used, violate, void, vow, vulnerable, warm, weak, weary, weepy, whimper, whispering, widow, withdrawn, woe, worry, wreckage, worthless, zombie

day bleeds into night
it all starts and ends the same
— rise says the moon

poem

her pain is so great that
she can't shake it, focus
or think of anything else

on these days
she can feel herself fading
slipping away from this life
just as her father did

poem

a series of bad days
if only she could see
past the pain
beyond the crashing waves

if only she could sleep
through
just one night

if only...

poem

this puddle of grief
strains her soul
and still she fights
surviving another day

poem

she absorbs her losses
never fully healing
their remains are
a part of her now
a piece of her existence
shaping her into a
stronger
BRAVER
version of herself

poem

I will
get
through
this!

no matter how dark the night
in the morning new light filters in
covering every corner of the darkness

poem

losing you was the start
of the shedding of my skin
nothing is the same

poem

a howling thunder
fall of the mighty redwood
death of my father

poem

sometimes i crawl down
into my skin, losing touch
i feel your presence

poem

I am taking
my time to
grieve.

the smallest trigger
a song, a smell, an instant
where time can stand still

poem

beside him she waits
hand in hand, her eyes close off
it all slips away

poem

morning after thoughts
in just a blink of an eye
she was fatherless

poem

why is it that where
your story ends, mine unravels
spitting new chapters?

poem

a double-edged sword
plunged into my heart, the night
you took your last breath

poem

In my
grief
I have
changed.

deafening silence
deep down she wants to scream
her eyes waste away

poem

i must wake up now
push my dreams aside; realize
that you really did die

poem

i feel you are near
strong, loving arms holding me
far away dreaming

poem

grief lives in our veins
a tornado; ripping apart
everything it comes across

poem

i don't want to move on
for fear it will take me further
from your living voice

poem

grief rises and falls
moving through peaks and valleys
unshakeable force

poem

all this hurt inside
moments of screaming and purging
bursting with anger

poem

It's okay
to be
angry!

the reality
burns the inside of my eyelids
— you are gone for good

poem

i dread the daylight
but i do not fear the dark
you'll visit me in my dreams

poem

smelling nostalgia
looking for familiar faces
you are everywhere

poem

I'm
discovering
my strengths
within
myself.

this pain weakens her
she lives your last breath over
and over again

poem

darkness lurks inside
distorted battles with my thoughts
weeping willow tree

poem

my thoughts are shifty
moving from dark to light corners
— late night dialogue

poem

depths of depression
i'm counting the days until
i see you again

poem

after the storm breaks
the sorrow will lift and joy
will return again

poem

I can
still see the
love in
the world.

failing to sleep
your lifeless body still haunts me
it rips me in two

a tree out of season
all my leaves are stripped away
i am left open

poem

one day you'll be okay
but right now, you need to sit
and make room for grief

poem

since you left this place
i have been trying to find
ways back to myself

poem

as the years pile up
there are moments where it's still
difficult to breathe

poem

this grief is unkind
unshakeable; dreadfully patient
an invisible burden

poem

crushing tsunami
is this the dark side of love
pressing down on me?

poem

I choose love, I choose to heal.

dear heart take your time
dabble into the darkness but
cycle back to the light

poem

lifted foundations
death separated us but
love bonds us forever

poem

Today
is for
healing.

out of focus lens
a clock of sadness that never lifts
life of a griever

poem

i live for the nights
where semi lucid dreaming
brings you back to me

poem

love and grief grow
from the same seed, hand in hand
an eternal bond

poem

time does not heal wounds
she just learns to move along
deepened, ebb and flow

poem

you've been beaten down
unwind, stop and just breathe
take time, rest your soul

poem

she's healing, although
the memories still haunt her
one, swift last breath

poem

in life there are waves
painful moments that change you
cascading rhythms

poem

life altered by pain
unconditional self-love
pathway to healing

poem

Happiness
and grief
can
coexist.

my heart is big enough
to hold everything I've ever
loved in every season

poem

you can fall apart
tonight and still rise
like a phoenix tomorrow

poem

there is still a light
ready to pour through you
don't you dare give up

poem

unresolved questions
numbness dances with disbelief
make space for this grief

poem

let those tears release
the finest bit of sorrow
lift the weight from your chest

poem

no timeline in sight
bittersweet and beautiful
she rebuild herself

poem

we don't get over loss
the hardening blow just
softens over time

poem

she knows great sadness
failure, defeat, but she also
knows resilience

poem

Write a letter to them

It's okay
to feel
however
I feel.

Weekly Reflection

WEEK: ___________

WHAT I'M FEELING RIGHT NOW ?

____
____
____
____
____
____
____
____

I'M REALLY MISSING...	I'M HAVING A HARD TIME WITH...

I CAN SHOW COMPASSION TO MYSELF BY....

☐ ____
☐ ____
☐

THINGS I'M GRATEFUL FOR...	GOOD THINGS ABOUT THIS WEEK...	SOMETHING THAT MADE ME SMILE...

Weekly Reflection

WEEK: _______________

WHAT I'M FEELING RIGHT NOW ?

____

____

____

____

____

____

____

____

I'M REALLY MISSING...	I'M HAVING A HARD TIME WITH...

I CAN SHOW COMPASSION TO MYSELF BY....

☐ ____

☐ ____

☐

THINGS I'M GRATEFUL FOR...	GOOD THINGS ABOUT THIS WEEK...	SOMETHING THAT MADE ME SMILE...

Weekly Reflection

WEEK: _______________

WHAT I'M FEELING RIGHT NOW ?

____
____
____
____
____
____
____
____

I'M REALLY MISSING...	I'M HAVING A HARD TIME WITH...

I CAN SHOW COMPASSION TO MYSELF BY....

☐ ____
☐ ____
☐

THINGS I'M GRATEFUL FOR...	GOOD THINGS ABOUT THIS WEEK...	SOMETHING THAT MADE ME SMILE...

Weekly Reflection

WEEK: _______________

WHAT I'M FEELING RIGHT NOW ?

____
____
____
____
____
____
____
____

I'M REALLY MISSING...	I'M HAVING A HARD TIME WITH...

I CAN SHOW COMPASSION TO MYSELF BY....

☐ ______________________________________
☐ ______________________________________
☐ ______________________________________

THINGS I'M GRATEFUL FOR...	GOOD THINGS ABOUT THIS WEEK...	SOMETHING THAT MADE ME SMILE...

Weekly Reflection

WEEK: _______________

WHAT I'M FEELING RIGHT NOW ?

____

____

____

____

____

____

____

____

____

I'M REALLY MISSING...	I'M HAVING A HARD TIME WITH...

I CAN SHOW COMPASSION TO MYSELF BY....

☐ ____

☐ ____

☐

THINGS I'M GRATEFUL FOR...	GOOD THINGS ABOUT THIS WEEK...	SOMETHING THAT MADE ME SMILE...

Weekly Reflection

WEEK: _______________

WHAT I'M FEELING RIGHT NOW ?

____
____
____
____
____
____
____
____
____

I'M REALLY MISSING...	I'M HAVING A HARD TIME WITH...

I CAN SHOW COMPASSION TO MYSELF BY....

☐ ____

☐ ____

☐

THINGS I'M GRATEFUL FOR...	GOOD THINGS ABOUT THIS WEEK...	SOMETHING THAT MADE ME SMILE...

Weekly Reflection

WEEK: _______________

WHAT I'M FEELING RIGHT NOW ?

____
____
____
____
____
____
____
____
____

I'M REALLY MISSING...	I'M HAVING A HARD TIME WITH...

I CAN SHOW COMPASSION TO MYSELF BY....

☐ ____
☐ ____
☐

THINGS I'M GRATEFUL FOR...	GOOD THINGS ABOUT THIS WEEK...	SOMETHING THAT MADE ME SMILE...

Weekly Reflection

WEEK: _______________

WHAT I'M FEELING RIGHT NOW ?

____

____

____

____

____

____

____

____

____

I'M REALLY MISSING...	I'M HAVING A HARD TIME WITH...

I CAN SHOW COMPASSION TO MYSELF BY....

☐ ____

☐ ____

☐ ____

THINGS I'M GRATEFUL FOR...	GOOD THINGS ABOUT THIS WEEK...	SOMETHING THAT MADE ME SMILE...

Weekly Reflection

WEEK: _______________

WHAT I'M FEELING RIGHT NOW ?

____
____
____
____
____
____
____
____
____

I'M REALLY MISSING...	I'M HAVING A HARD TIME WITH...

I CAN SHOW COMPASSION TO MYSELF BY....

☐ ____

☐ ____

☐

THINGS I'M GRATEFUL FOR...	GOOD THINGS ABOUT THIS WEEK...	SOMETHING THAT MADE ME SMILE...

Weekly Reflection

WEEK: ______________

WHAT I'M FEELING RIGHT NOW ?

____

____

____

____

____

____

____

____

____

I'M REALLY MISSING...	I'M HAVING A HARD TIME WITH...

I CAN SHOW COMPASSION TO MYSELF BY....

☐ ____

☐ ____

☐

THINGS I'M GRATEFUL FOR...	GOOD THINGS ABOUT THIS WEEK...	SOMETHING THAT MADE ME SMILE...

Weekly Reflection

WEEK: _______________

WHAT I'M FEELING RIGHT NOW ?

I'M REALLY MISSING...	I'M HAVING A HARD TIME WITH...

I CAN SHOW COMPASSION TO MYSELF BY....

☐ ____

☐ ____

☐

THINGS I'M GRATEFUL FOR...	GOOD THINGS ABOUT THIS WEEK...	SOMETHING THAT MADE ME SMILE...

Weekly Reflection

WEEK: _____________

WHAT I'M FEELING RIGHT NOW ?

____

____

____

____

____

____

____

____

____

I'M REALLY MISSING...	I'M HAVING A HARD TIME WITH...

I CAN SHOW COMPASSION TO MYSELF BY....

☐ _______________________________________

☐ _______________________________________

☐ _______________________________________

THINGS I'M GRATEFUL FOR...	GOOD THINGS ABOUT THIS WEEK...	SOMETHING THAT MADE ME SMILE...

Weekly Reflection

WEEK: _______________

WHAT I'M FEELING RIGHT NOW ?

I'M REALLY MISSING...	I'M HAVING A HARD TIME WITH...

I CAN SHOW COMPASSION TO MYSELF BY....

☐ ____

☐ ____

☐

THINGS I'M GRATEFUL FOR...	GOOD THINGS ABOUT THIS WEEK...	SOMETHING THAT MADE ME SMILE...

Weekly Reflection

WEEK: _______________

WHAT I'M FEELING RIGHT NOW ?

____
____
____
____
____
____
____
____
____

I'M REALLY MISSING...	I'M HAVING A HARD TIME WITH...

I CAN SHOW COMPASSION TO MYSELF BY....

☐ ____
☐ ____
☐ ____

THINGS I'M GRATEFUL FOR...	GOOD THINGS ABOUT THIS WEEK...	SOMETHING THAT MADE ME SMILE...

Weekly Reflection

WEEK: _______________

WHAT I'M FEELING RIGHT NOW ?

____
____
____
____
____
____
____
____

I'M REALLY MISSING...	I'M HAVING A HARD TIME WITH...

I CAN SHOW COMPASSION TO MYSELF BY....

☐ ____

☐ ____

☐

THINGS I'M GRATEFUL FOR...	GOOD THINGS ABOUT THIS WEEK...	SOMETHING THAT MADE ME SMILE...

Weekly Reflection

WEEK: ______________

WHAT I'M FEELING RIGHT NOW?

____
____
____
____
____
____
____
____

I'M REALLY MISSING...	I'M HAVING A HARD TIME WITH...

I CAN SHOW COMPASSION TO MYSELF BY....

- ☐ ____
- ☐ ____
- ☐ ____

THINGS I'M GRATEFUL FOR...	GOOD THINGS ABOUT THIS WEEK...	SOMETHING THAT MADE ME SMILE...

Weekly Reflection

WEEK: _____________

WHAT I'M FEELING RIGHT NOW ?

____
____
____
____
____
____
____
____

I'M REALLY MISSING...	I'M HAVING A HARD TIME WITH...

I CAN SHOW COMPASSION TO MYSELF BY....

☐ ____

☐ ____

☐

THINGS I'M GRATEFUL FOR...	GOOD THINGS ABOUT THIS WEEK...	SOMETHING THAT MADE ME SMILE...

Weekly Reflection

WEEK: ___________

WHAT I'M FEELING RIGHT NOW ?

____
____
____
____
____
____
____
____

I'M REALLY MISSING...	I'M HAVING A HARD TIME WITH...

I CAN SHOW COMPASSION TO MYSELF BY....

☐ _______________________________________
☐ _______________________________________
☐ _______________________________________

THINGS I'M GRATEFUL FOR...	GOOD THINGS ABOUT THIS WEEK...	SOMETHING THAT MADE ME SMILE...

Weekly Reflection

WEEK: _____________

WHAT I'M FEELING RIGHT NOW ?

____
____
____
____
____
____
____
____
____

I'M REALLY MISSING...	I'M HAVING A HARD TIME WITH...

I CAN SHOW COMPASSION TO MYSELF BY....

☐ ____
☐ ____
☐

THINGS I'M GRATEFUL FOR...	GOOD THINGS ABOUT THIS WEEK...	SOMETHING THAT MADE ME SMILE...

Weekly Reflection

WEEK: _______________

WHAT I'M FEELING RIGHT NOW ?

____
____
____
____
____
____
____
____
____

I'M REALLY MISSING...	I'M HAVING A HARD TIME WITH...

I CAN SHOW COMPASSION TO MYSELF BY....

☐ _______________________________________
☐ _______________________________________
☐ _______________________________________

THINGS I'M GRATEFUL FOR...	GOOD THINGS ABOUT THIS WEEK...	SOMETHING THAT MADE ME SMILE...

Weekly Reflection

WEEK: _______________

WHAT I'M FEELING RIGHT NOW ?

____
____
____
____
____
____
____
____

I'M REALLY MISSING...	I'M HAVING A HARD TIME WITH...

I CAN SHOW COMPASSION TO MYSELF BY....

☐ ____
☐ ____
☐ ____

THINGS I'M GRATEFUL FOR...	GOOD THINGS ABOUT THIS WEEK...	SOMETHING THAT MADE ME SMILE...

Weekly Reflection

WEEK: ______________

WHAT I'M FEELING RIGHT NOW ?

____
____
____
____
____
____
____
____

I'M REALLY MISSING...	I'M HAVING A HARD TIME WITH...

I CAN SHOW COMPASSION TO MYSELF BY....

- ☐ _______________________________________
- ☐ _______________________________________
- ☐

THINGS I'M GRATEFUL FOR...	GOOD THINGS ABOUT THIS WEEK...	SOMETHING THAT MADE ME SMILE...

Weekly Reflection

WEEK: _____________

WHAT I'M FEELING RIGHT NOW ?

____

____

____

____

____

____

____

____

I'M REALLY MISSING...	I'M HAVING A HARD TIME WITH...

I CAN SHOW COMPASSION TO MYSELF BY....

☐ ____

☐ ____

☐

THINGS I'M GRATEFUL FOR...	GOOD THINGS ABOUT THIS WEEK...	SOMETHING THAT MADE ME SMILE...

Weekly Reflection

WEEK: __________

WHAT I'M FEELING RIGHT NOW ?

____

____

____

____

____

____

____

____

____

I'M REALLY MISSING...	I'M HAVING A HARD TIME WITH...

I CAN SHOW COMPASSION TO MYSELF BY....

☐ ____

☐ ____

☐

THINGS I'M GRATEFUL FOR...	GOOD THINGS ABOUT THIS WEEK...	SOMETHING THAT MADE ME SMILE...

Weekly Reflection

WEEK: ______________

WHAT I'M FEELING RIGHT NOW?

____

____

____

____

____

____

____

____

____

I'M REALLY MISSING...	I'M HAVING A HARD TIME WITH...

I CAN SHOW COMPASSION TO MYSELF BY....

☐ ____

☐ ____

☐

THINGS I'M GRATEFUL FOR...	GOOD THINGS ABOUT THIS WEEK...	SOMETHING THAT MADE ME SMILE...

Weekly Reflection

WEEK: ________

WHAT I'M FEELING RIGHT NOW ?

____
____
____
____
____
____
____
____
____

I'M REALLY MISSING...	I'M HAVING A HARD TIME WITH...

I CAN SHOW COMPASSION TO MYSELF BY....

☐ ____
☐ ____
☐

THINGS I'M GRATEFUL FOR...	GOOD THINGS ABOUT THIS WEEK...	SOMETHING THAT MADE ME SMILE...

Weekly Reflection

WEEK: _______________

____

____

____

____

____

____

____

____

I'M REALLY MISSING...	I'M HAVING A HARD TIME WITH...

I CAN SHOW COMPASSION TO MYSELF BY....

☐ ____

☐ ____

☐

THINGS I'M GRATEFUL FOR...	GOOD THINGS ABOUT THIS WEEK...	SOMETHING THAT MADE ME SMILE...

Weekly Reflection

WEEK: _______________

WHAT I'M FEELING RIGHT NOW ?

____
____
____
____
____
____
____
____
____

I'M REALLY MISSING...	I'M HAVING A HARD TIME WITH...

I CAN SHOW COMPASSION TO MYSELF BY....

☐ ____
☐ ____
☐ ____

THINGS I'M GRATEFUL FOR...	GOOD THINGS ABOUT THIS WEEK...	SOMETHING THAT MADE ME SMILE...

Weekly Reflection

WEEK: _____________

WHAT I'M FEELING RIGHT NOW ?

____
____
____
____
____
____
____
____
____

I'M REALLY MISSING...	I'M HAVING A HARD TIME WITH...

I CAN SHOW COMPASSION TO MYSELF BY....

☐ ____
☐ ____
☐ ____

THINGS I'M GRATEFUL FOR...	GOOD THINGS ABOUT THIS WEEK...	SOMETHING THAT MADE ME SMILE...

Weekly Reflection

WEEK: _______________

WHAT I'M FEELING RIGHT NOW ?

____
____
____
____
____
____
____
____

I'M REALLY MISSING...	I'M HAVING A HARD TIME WITH...

I CAN SHOW COMPASSION TO MYSELF BY....

☐ _______________________________________
☐ _______________________________________
☐

THINGS I'M GRATEFUL FOR...	GOOD THINGS ABOUT THIS WEEK...	SOMETHING THAT MADE ME SMILE...

Weekly Reflection

WEEK: _______________

WHAT I'M FEELING RIGHT NOW ?

____

____

____

____

____

____

____

____

____

I'M REALLY MISSING...	I'M HAVING A HARD TIME WITH...

I CAN SHOW COMPASSION TO MYSELF BY....

☐ ____

☐ ____

☐

THINGS I'M GRATEFUL FOR...	GOOD THINGS ABOUT THIS WEEK...	SOMETHING THAT MADE ME SMILE...

Weekly Reflection

WEEK: ___________

WHAT I'M FEELING RIGHT NOW ?

____
____
____
____
____
____
____
____
____

<table>
<tr><td>I'M REALLY MISSING...</td><td>I'M HAVING A HARD TIME WITH...</td></tr>
<tr><td>

</td><td>

</td></tr>
</table>

I CAN SHOW COMPASSION TO MYSELF BY....

☐ _______________________________________
☐ _______________________________________
☐ _______________________________________

THINGS I'M GRATEFUL FOR...	GOOD THINGS ABOUT THIS WEEK...	SOMETHING THAT MADE ME SMILE...

Weekly Reflection

WEEK: ___________

WHAT I'M FEELING RIGHT NOW ?

____

____

____

____

____

____

____

____

I'M REALLY MISSING...	I'M HAVING A HARD TIME WITH...

I CAN SHOW COMPASSION TO MYSELF BY....

☐ ____

☐ ____

☐

THINGS I'M GRATEFUL FOR...	GOOD THINGS ABOUT THIS WEEK...	SOMETHING THAT MADE ME SMILE...

Weekly Reflection

WEEK: _______________

WHAT I'M FEELING RIGHT NOW?

____

____

____

____

____

____

____

____

I'M REALLY MISSING...	I'M HAVING A HARD TIME WITH...

I CAN SHOW COMPASSION TO MYSELF BY....

☐ ____

☐ ____

☐

THINGS I'M GRATEFUL FOR...	GOOD THINGS ABOUT THIS WEEK...	SOMETHING THAT MADE ME SMILE...

Weekly Reflection

WEEK: _____________

WHAT I'M FEELING RIGHT NOW ?

____
____
____
____
____
____
____
____

I'M REALLY MISSING...	I'M HAVING A HARD TIME WITH...

I CAN SHOW COMPASSION TO MYSELF BY....

☐ ____
☐ ____
☐

THINGS I'M GRATEFUL FOR...	GOOD THINGS ABOUT THIS WEEK...	SOMETHING THAT MADE ME SMILE...

Weekly Reflection

WEEK: _______________

WHAT I'M FEELING RIGHT NOW ?

____

____

____

____

____

____

____

____

____

I'M REALLY MISSING...	I'M HAVING A HARD TIME WITH...

I CAN SHOW COMPASSION TO MYSELF BY....

☐ ____

☐ ____

☐

THINGS I'M GRATEFUL FOR...	GOOD THINGS ABOUT THIS WEEK...	SOMETHING THAT MADE ME SMILE...

Weekly Reflection

WEEK: _______________

WHAT I'M FEELING RIGHT NOW ?

____

____

____

____

____

____

____

____

____

I'M REALLY MISSING...	I'M HAVING A HARD TIME WITH...

I CAN SHOW COMPASSION TO MYSELF BY....

☐ ____

☐ ____

☐

THINGS I'M GRATEFUL FOR...	GOOD THINGS ABOUT THIS WEEK...	SOMETHING THAT MADE ME SMILE...

Weekly Reflection

WEEK: _______________

WHAT I'M FEELING RIGHT NOW ?

____
____
____
____
____
____
____
____
____

I'M REALLY MISSING...	I'M HAVING A HARD TIME WITH...

I CAN SHOW COMPASSION TO MYSELF BY....

☐ ____
☐ ____
☐

THINGS I'M GRATEFUL FOR...	GOOD THINGS ABOUT THIS WEEK...	SOMETHING THAT MADE ME SMILE...

Weekly Reflection

WEEK: _______________

WHAT I'M FEELING RIGHT NOW ?

____

____

____

____

____

____

____

____

I'M REALLY MISSING...	I'M HAVING A HARD TIME WITH...

I CAN SHOW COMPASSION TO MYSELF BY....

☐ ____

☐ ____

☐ ____

THINGS I'M GRATEFUL FOR...	GOOD THINGS ABOUT THIS WEEK...	SOMETHING THAT MADE ME SMILE...

Weekly Reflection

WEEK: _____________

WHAT I'M FEELING RIGHT NOW ?

____
____
____
____
____
____
____
____

I'M REALLY MISSING...	I'M HAVING A HARD TIME WITH...

I CAN SHOW COMPASSION TO MYSELF BY....

☐ ____

☐ ____

☐

THINGS I'M GRATEFUL FOR...	GOOD THINGS ABOUT THIS WEEK...	SOMETHING THAT MADE ME SMILE...

Weekly Reflection

WEEK: _______________

WHAT I'M FEELING RIGHT NOW ?

____

____

____

____

____

____

____

____

I'M REALLY MISSING...	I'M HAVING A HARD TIME WITH...

I CAN SHOW COMPASSION TO MYSELF BY....

☐ ____

☐ ____

☐

THINGS I'M GRATEFUL FOR...	GOOD THINGS ABOUT THIS WEEK...	SOMETHING THAT MADE ME SMILE...

Weekly Reflection

WEEK: ________________

WHAT I'M FEELING RIGHT NOW ?

____
____
____
____
____
____
____
____

I'M REALLY MISSING...	I'M HAVING A HARD TIME WITH...

I CAN SHOW COMPASSION TO MYSELF BY....

☐ ____
☐ ____
☐ ____

THINGS I'M GRATEFUL FOR...	GOOD THINGS ABOUT THIS WEEK...	SOMETHING THAT MADE ME SMILE...

Weekly Reflection

WEEK: _____________

WHAT I'M FEELING RIGHT NOW ?

____
____
____
____
____
____
____
____
____

I'M REALLY MISSING...	I'M HAVING A HARD TIME WITH...

I CAN SHOW COMPASSION TO MYSELF BY....

☐ ____

☐ ____

☐

THINGS I'M GRATEFUL FOR...	GOOD THINGS ABOUT THIS WEEK...	SOMETHING THAT MADE ME SMILE...

Weekly Reflection

WEEK: _______________

WHAT I'M FEELING RIGHT NOW ?

____
____
____
____
____
____
____
____
____

I'M REALLY MISSING...	I'M HAVING A HARD TIME WITH...

I CAN SHOW COMPASSION TO MYSELF BY....

☐ ____
☐ ____
☐

THINGS I'M GRATEFUL FOR...	GOOD THINGS ABOUT THIS WEEK...	SOMETHING THAT MADE ME SMILE...

Weekly Reflection

WEEK: _______________

WHAT I'M FEELING RIGHT NOW ?

____
____
____
____
____
____
____
____

I'M REALLY MISSING...	I'M HAVING A HARD TIME WITH...

I CAN SHOW COMPASSION TO MYSELF BY....

☐ ____
☐ ____
☐

THINGS I'M GRATEFUL FOR...	GOOD THINGS ABOUT THIS WEEK...	SOMETHING THAT MADE ME SMILE...

Weekly Reflection

WEEK: ______________

WHAT I'M FEELING RIGHT NOW ?

____

____

____

____

____

____

____

____

____

I'M REALLY MISSING...	I'M HAVING A HARD TIME WITH...

I CAN SHOW COMPASSION TO MYSELF BY....

☐ ____

☐ ____

☐ ____

THINGS I'M GRATEFUL FOR...	GOOD THINGS ABOUT THIS WEEK...	SOMETHING THAT MADE ME SMILE...

Weekly Reflection

WEEK: _______________

WHAT I'M FEELING RIGHT NOW ?

____
____
____
____
____
____
____
____
____

I'M REALLY MISSING...	I'M HAVING A HARD TIME WITH...

I CAN SHOW COMPASSION TO MYSELF BY....

☐ ____
☐ ____
☐

THINGS I'M GRATEFUL FOR...	GOOD THINGS ABOUT THIS WEEK...	SOMETHING THAT MADE ME SMILE...

Weekly Reflection

WEEK: ______________

I'M REALLY MISSING...	I'M HAVING A HARD TIME WITH...

I CAN SHOW COMPASSION TO MYSELF BY....

☐ ______________________________________

☐ ______________________________________

☐

THINGS I'M GRATEFUL FOR...	GOOD THINGS ABOUT THIS WEEK...	SOMETHING THAT MADE ME SMILE...

Weekly Reflection

WEEK: _______________

WHAT I'M FEELING RIGHT NOW ?

____

____

____

____

____

____

____

____

____

I'M REALLY MISSING...	I'M HAVING A HARD TIME WITH...

I CAN SHOW COMPASSION TO MYSELF BY....

☐ ____

☐ ____

☐

THINGS I'M GRATEFUL FOR...	GOOD THINGS ABOUT THIS WEEK...	SOMETHING THAT MADE ME SMILE...

Weekly Reflection

WEEK: ________________

WHAT I'M FEELING RIGHT NOW ?

____
____
____
____
____
____
____
____
____

I'M REALLY MISSING...	I'M HAVING A HARD TIME WITH...

I CAN SHOW COMPASSION TO MYSELF BY....

☐ ____

☐ ____

☐

THINGS I'M GRATEFUL FOR...	GOOD THINGS ABOUT THIS WEEK...	SOMETHING THAT MADE ME SMILE...

Weekly Reflection

WEEK: _______________

WHAT I'M FEELING RIGHT NOW ?

____

____

____

____

____

____

____

____

I'M REALLY MISSING...	I'M HAVING A HARD TIME WITH...

I CAN SHOW COMPASSION TO MYSELF BY....

☐ ____

☐ ____

☐

THINGS I'M GRATEFUL FOR...	GOOD THINGS ABOUT THIS WEEK...	SOMETHING THAT MADE ME SMILE...

Weekly Reflection

WEEK: ______________

> WHAT I'M FEELING RIGHT NOW ?

____

____

____

____

____

____

____

____

I'M REALLY MISSING...	I'M HAVING A HARD TIME WITH...

> I CAN SHOW COMPASSION TO MYSELF BY....

☐ _______________________________________

☐ _______________________________________

☐ _______________________________________

THINGS I'M GRATEFUL FOR...	GOOD THINGS ABOUT THIS WEEK...	SOMETHING THAT MADE ME SMILE...

I am ready
for this

new

chapter.

Journaling

Writing in a journal can be one of the most powerful ways to cope and work towards your healing. Journaling encourages introspection, which is important in accepting loss.

One of the best parts about journaling is that there is no right or wrong way to do it. You can write about how you feel and why you feel that way. Remember that you're writing for yourself, no one else. Truly, take this time to let go of all that you're feeling. Sometimes the words will flow out of you with little thought, and other times you might feel stuck, and that's okay. Reading back on what you wrote last time will often give you a starting point for your next entry. We all feel the need to make sense of the world around us. The death of a loved one shakes our foundations. It takes time to reorganize our beliefs and find hope for the future—but sometimes, journaling can be the first step in that journey.

Within the pages of this part of the book, allow yourself the freedom of complete self-expression.

- Try not to censor yourself. Write down everything that comes to mind. Don't worry about grammar and spelling.
- Journal writing is a creative expression. Give yourself permission to openly and honestly express yourself. If you are holding back out of fear that someone may find your journal, then try to keep it in a secure place.
- Attempt to put aside at least 5 to 10 minutes a day for journaling. Figure out what time of day is best for you. Consider writing in the morning to get all your worries, frustrations, and hopes for the day out of your system or to write in the evening to reflect on your day.
- Try not to view journal writing as a task. Rather, consider it an opportunity to learn about yourself and cope with everything you're going through.

Today, I'm having a hard time with…

journal

One thing I want to remember about them is…

journal

If I could go back in time, I would do this differently.

journal

I don't ever want to forget…

journal

Describe a memory with your loved one that makes you laugh.

journal

The hardest time of day is...

journal

I feel guilty when I think about...

journal

Here's how I've changed since my loved one has died.

journal

I feel most connected to my loved one when

journal

The pain
in my
heart will
heal.

One feeling I've felt coming up a lot lately is…

journal

Write about the events that lead up to your loved one's death.

journal

If I had one more day with my loved one...

journal

What comforts you during your time of grief?

journal

Write about where you feel your grief in your body.
Where does your grief stay?

journal

What well-meaning words have people said to you that have caused heartache and grief?

journal

Write about a time you have felt anger.

journal

How can I take care of myself physically while grieving.

journal

List ways you can be kind to yourself.

journal

I am
patient with
my healing
process.

Describe your loved one's personality.

journal

What emotions do you have that you wouldn't feel
comfortable sharing with others?

journal

Describe a memory with your loved one that makes you laugh.

journal

Describe a memory with your loved one that makes you cry.

journal

One feeling I've felt coming up a lot lately is…

journal

Where does your mind go when you let it wander?

journal

What is one thing you could try to make today easier on yourself?

journal

I need more of…

journal

I need less of…

journal

Do you feel comfortable asking for help? Why or why not?

journal

I feel most connected to my loved one when…

journal

One thing I wish I could do over with them is…

journal

If I could forgive them for something, it would be…

journal

If I could forgive myself for something, it would be…

journal

If you could tell your loved one about your day,
what would you tell them?

journal

How did your loved one make you feel?

journal

Write a mantra you can return to when you feel overwhelmed
by grief.

journal

What is something you wish your support system would understand?

journal

What songs make you think of them?

journal

Some of my grief triggers are...

journal

Make a list of a few different ways you can honor your
loved one or your loss.

journal

Here are five ways I can be compassionate with myself today…

journal

I am
moving
forward.

notes

notes

197

"I don't think of all the misery, but of all the beauty that remains."
– Anne Frank

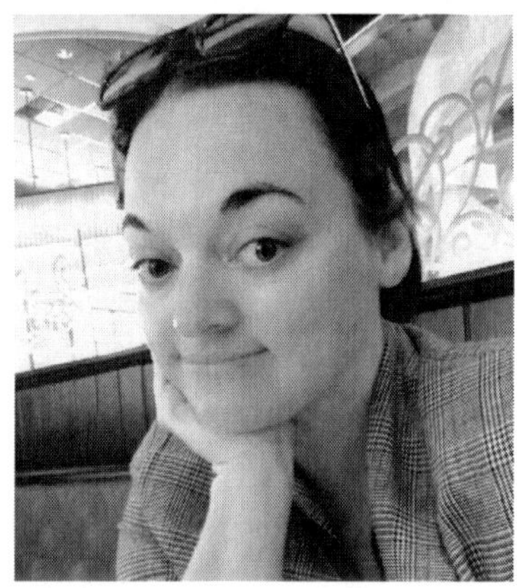

D.L. Heather is the pen name for poet, writer, and former music journalist Debra Heather. She has a B.A. in English and is the author of the inspirational poetry collections; Life Interrupted and Metamorphosis. Writing came into her life in her teens by way of therapy and the exploration of healing through journaling. Her writing is motivated by her experiences with childhood trauma, love, loss, healing, heartbreak, and self-discovery.

A private person by nature, she prefers to let her work speak for itself, in the way poetry allows her to. She hopes to inspire others and reinforce the fact that you are not alone. When she isn't writing in her studio, she enjoys traveling, reading, movies and gardening.

Connect with her @dlheatherpoetry
www.dlheatherbooks.net

First of all, thank you for purchasing this book. I know you could have picked any number of books to read, but you picked this one and for that I am extremely grateful. It would be really nice if you could share this book with your friends and family by posting to Instagram, Twitter or Facebook.

I'd like to hear from you and hope that you could take some time to leave a on Amazon.

Made in United States
North Haven, CT
10 November 2023